The Purpose of this Book.

Once clinicians and students learn how to read electrocardiograms and have participated in foundational classes in Basic and Advanced CPR, they are ready to confront the enemy – death.

CODE BLUE is the phrase everyone has become familiar with. The time when a patient's heart has either stopped or they have developed a rhythm that is life threatening. CARDIAC ARREST is the result of a rhythm that is no longer able to sustain life and when left untreated the patient will either sustain heart damage (MYOCARDIAL INFARCTION) or die.

This book provides some real life examples of cardiac arrest rhythms and some of the treatments for those rhythms to provide some practice opportunities to help prepare you for such patients.

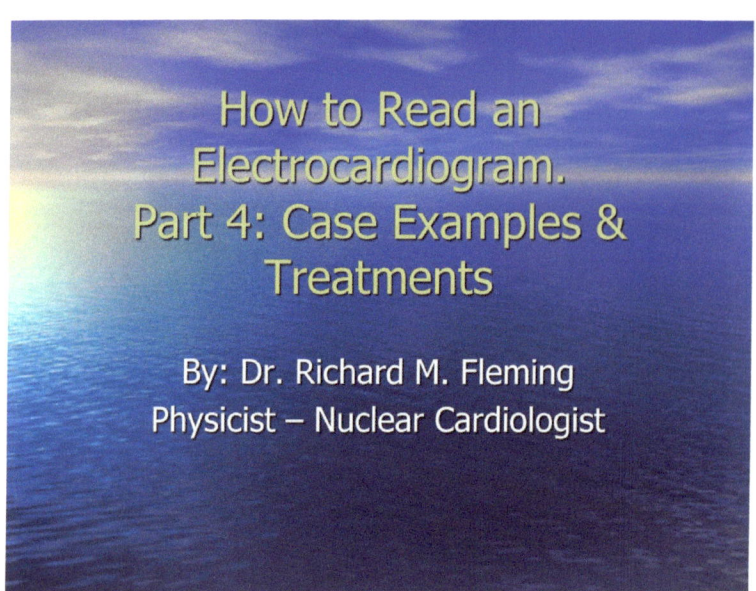
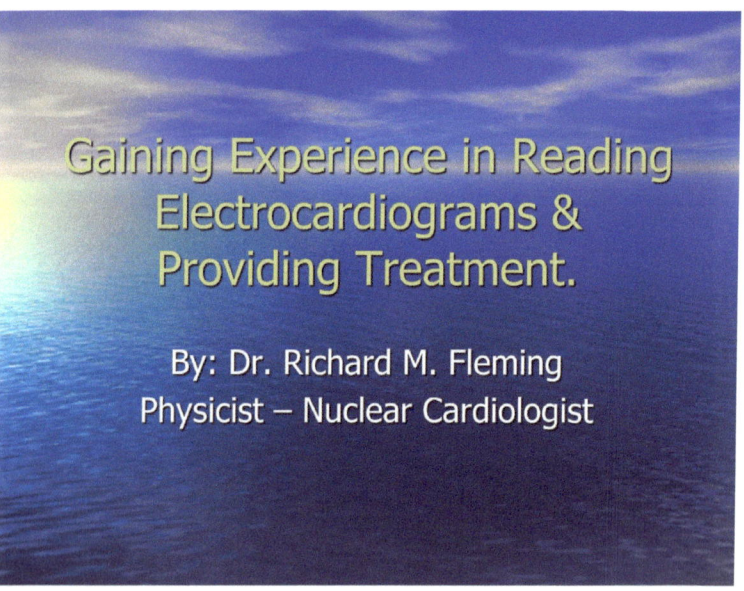

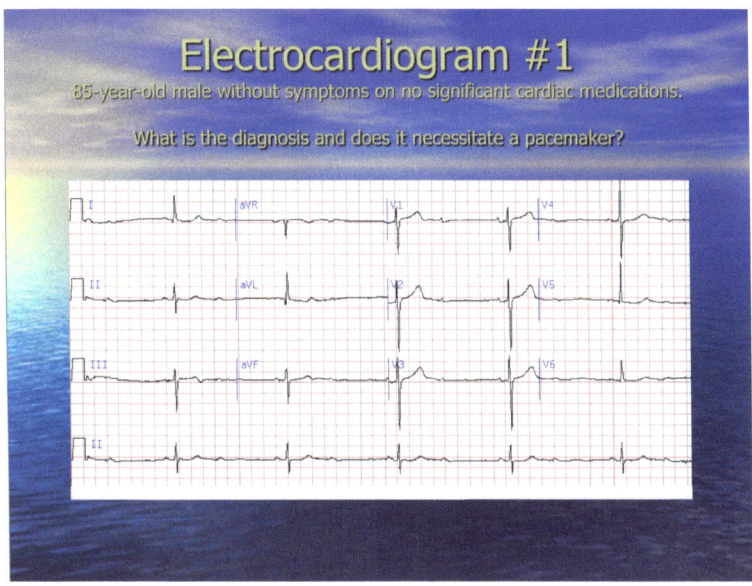

Sinus rhythm with 2:1 AV heart block. The ECG shows a brady dysrhythmia with non-conducted sinus P waves alternating with normally conducted P waves. It is not possible to reliably identify the point of block (nodal vs. infranodal) from this single ECG with 2:1 conduction. There is no evidence of acute inferior ischemia, either. The site of block could be proximal (in the AV node) or more distal, in the His-Purkinje system. In general, with 2:1 block, involvement of the AV node is favored by a narrow QRS complex and a prolonged PR interval, or by the presence of intermittent AV Wenckebach. Block (nfranodal) in the His-Purkinje system would be favored by a concomitant bundle branch block and/or with a PR interval of 160 ms or less. A possibly useful bedside diagnostic test for chronic 2:1 block (in the absence of active ischemia) would be to increase the sinus rate (mild exercise). A resumption of 1:1 conduction favors AV node block while worsening of block strongly favors infranodal disease. Pacemaker placement is indicated for symptomatic 2:1 block without reversible cause (e.g., drug effect) and generally for asymptomatic 2:1 block due to infranodal disease. An intracardiac His bundle electrocardiogram would definitively identify the site of block. This patient had intermittent 3:2 AV Wenckebach at other times, and then resumed 1:1 conduction on subsequent ECGs, consistent with AV node disease.

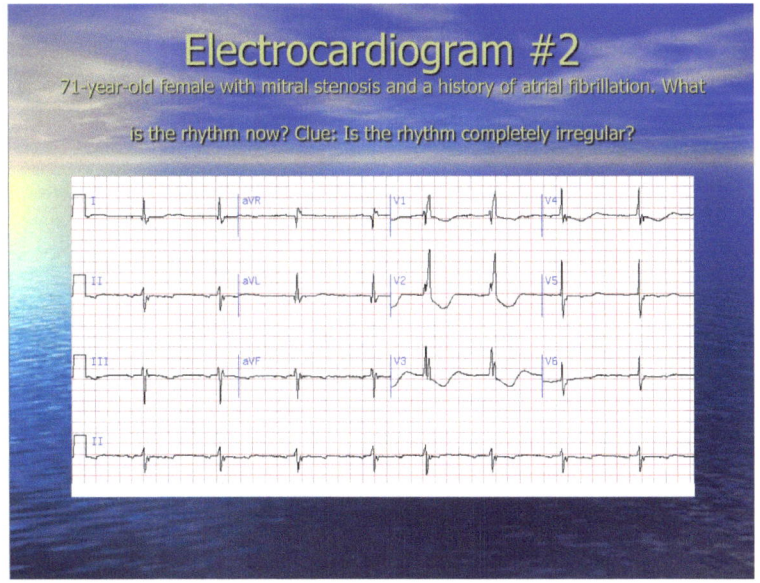

Rhythm: Ectopic atrial (non-sinus) tachycardia with 2:1 block and 3:2 AV Wenckebach (beats 4 and 5). Note the negative P waves in lead II indicating a non-sinus pacemaker. Other important abnormalities: right bundle branch block, left anterior fascicular block and a markedly prolonged QT(U) interval. This patient was on Digoxin and Quinidine. The evidence for Quinidine toxicity (assuming the serum potassium is normal and no other factors prolonging ventricular repolarization are identifiable) is the very long QT(U) interval best seen in V2-V5. This finding predisposes to torsade de pointes and may occur with "therapeutic" or "subtherapeutic" levels of Quinidine or other class 1A antiarrhythmic (antidysrhythmic) drugs. Atrial tachycardia with Mobitz I block also strongly raises the question of digitalis toxicity. With pure 2:1 AV block, it may be impossible from the surface ECG to tell if the non-conducted beats are due to nodal or infranodal block. The clue here centers on beats 4 and 5 where 3:2 Wenckebach is evident, indicating block in the AV node.

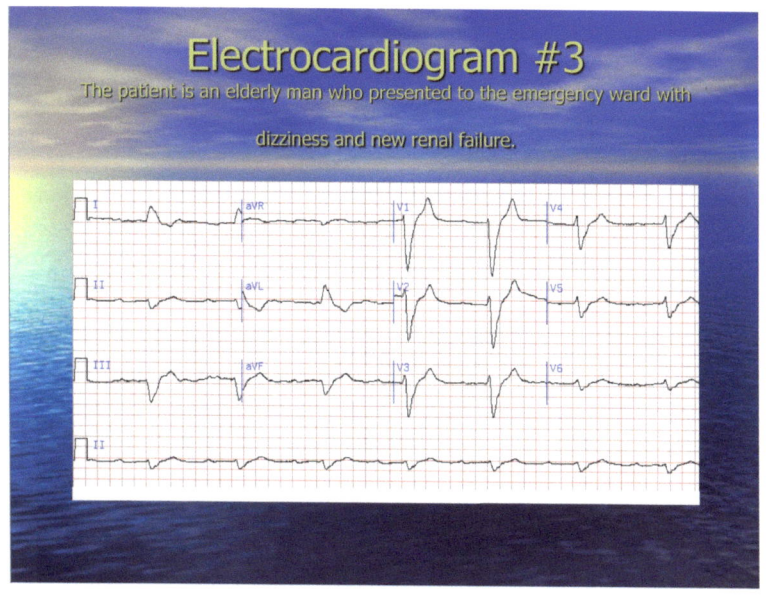

Diagnosis: Hyperkalemia (7.6 mEq/L) secondary to renal failure. The ECG demonstrates findings consistent with severe hyperkalemia - most importantly widening of the QRS complex. There is also peaking of the T waves with prolongation of the PR interval and flattening of the P waves. If the hyperkalemia is left untreated, the ECG will progress to a sinusoidal pattern and eventually asystole with subsequent hemodynamic collapse and death.

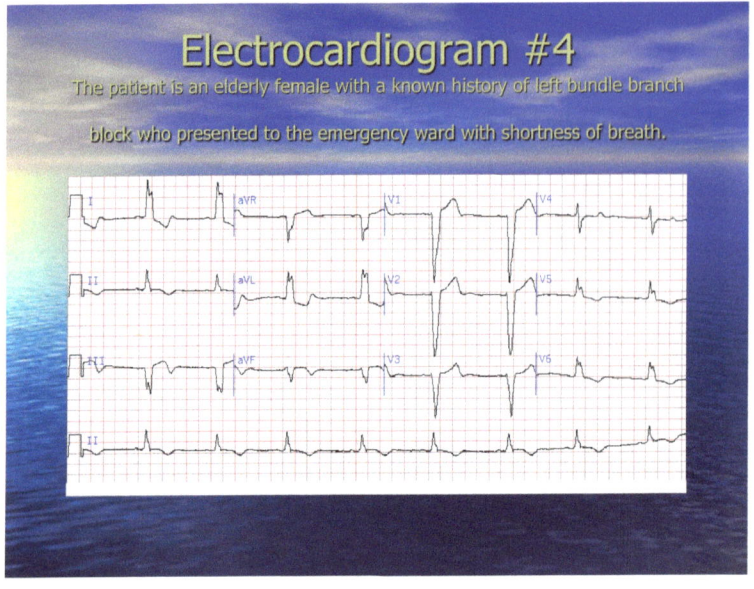

Diagnosis: Sinus bradycardia, left bundle branch block (LBBB) with primary ST-T wave changes. The ECG demonstrates a bundle (LBBB) morphology with primary biphasic and inverted T waves in leads 2, 3 and F. Uncomplicated bundle branch blocks should have "secondary" T wave changes. That is the ST-T waves should be opposite in direction to the major vector of the QRS. For example, if this ECG with LBBB was uncomplicated, the ST-T waves in the inferior leads would be upright. This patient has inverted T waves suggesting that a "primary" or ischemic process is evolving in the inferior distribution. She did in fact rule in for a myocardial infarction with a CK of 700 and 21% MB fraction. This example illustrates that ischemic ECG changes can sometimes be read despite the presence of a bundle branch block.

The Normal QRS Axis.

- By near-consensus, the normal QRS axis is defined as ranging from -30° to +90°.

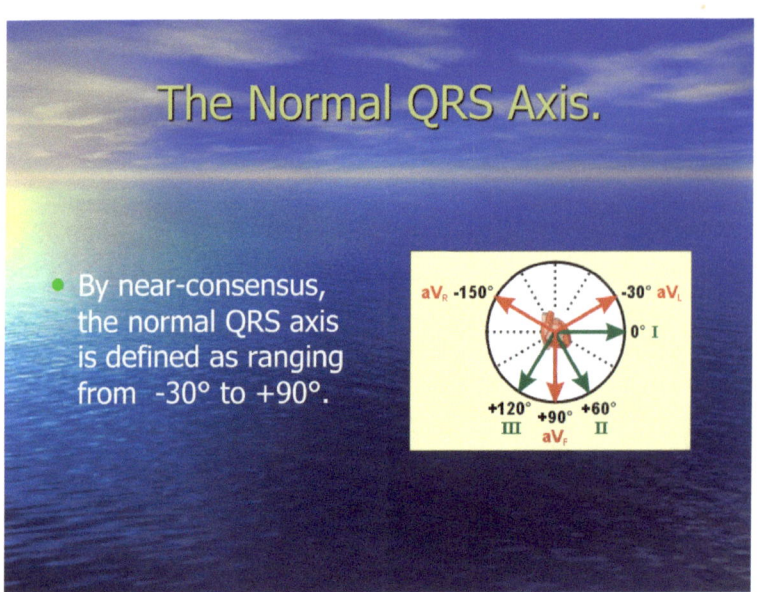

The QRS Axis

- -30° to -90° is referred to as a left axis deviation (LAD)

- +90° to +180° is referred to as a right axis deviation (RAD)

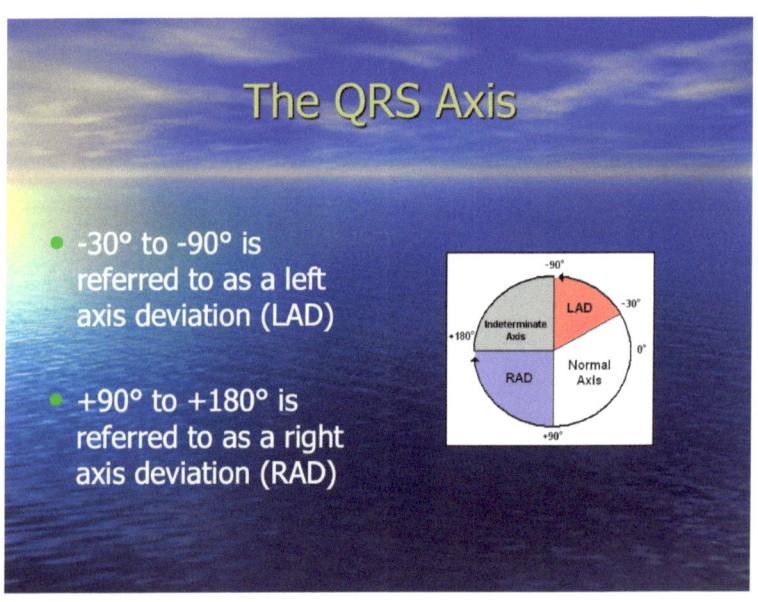

Normal (0°): QRS Axis

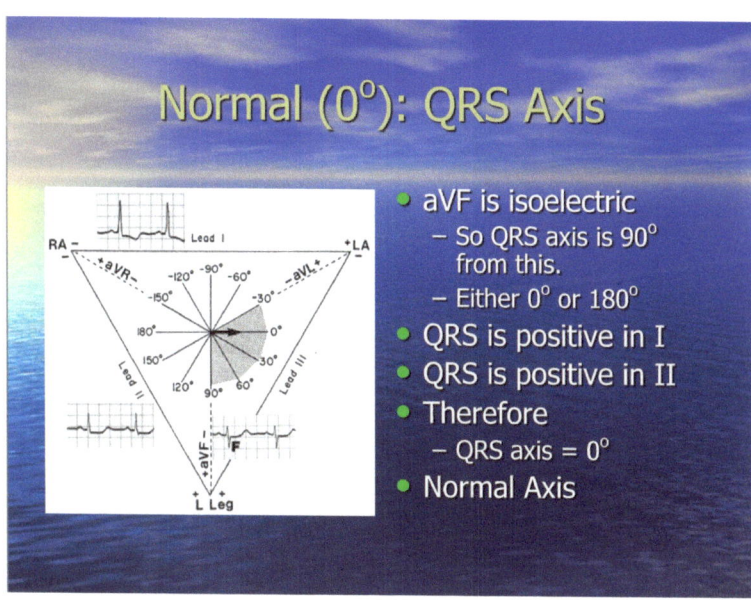

- aVF is isoelectric
  - So QRS axis is 90° from this.
  - Either 0° or 180°
- QRS is positive in I
- QRS is positive in II
- Therefore
  - QRS axis = 0°
- Normal Axis

LAD (-60°): aVR is isoelectric.

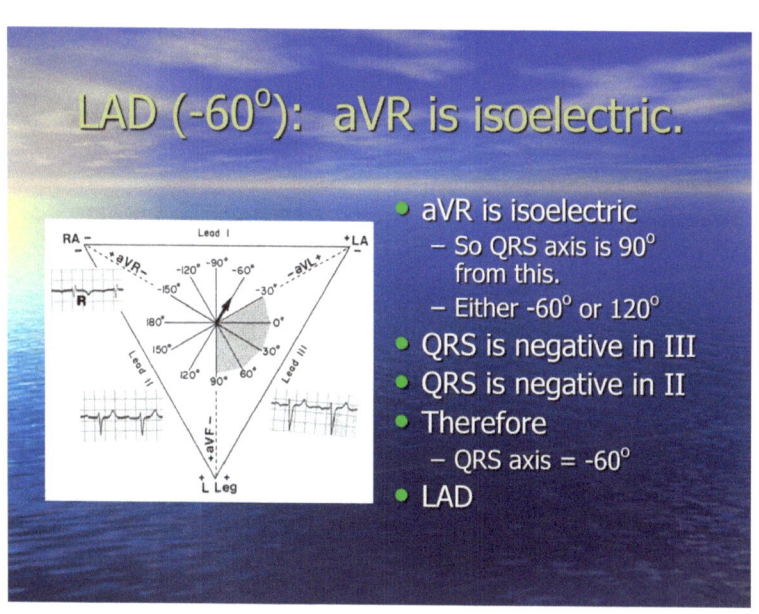

- aVR is isoelectric
  - So QRS axis is 90° from this.
  - Either -60° or 120°
- QRS is negative in III
- QRS is negative in II
- Therefore
  - QRS axis = -60°
- LAD

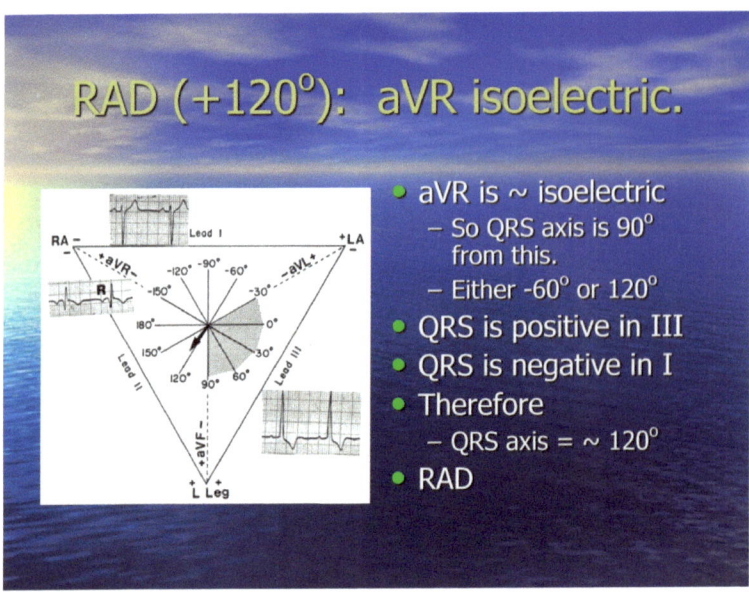

RAD (+120°): aVR isoelectric.

- aVR is ~ isoelectric
  - So QRS axis is 90° from this.
  - Either -60° or 120°
- QRS is positive in III
- QRS is negative in I
- Therefore
  - QRS axis = ~ 120°
- RAD

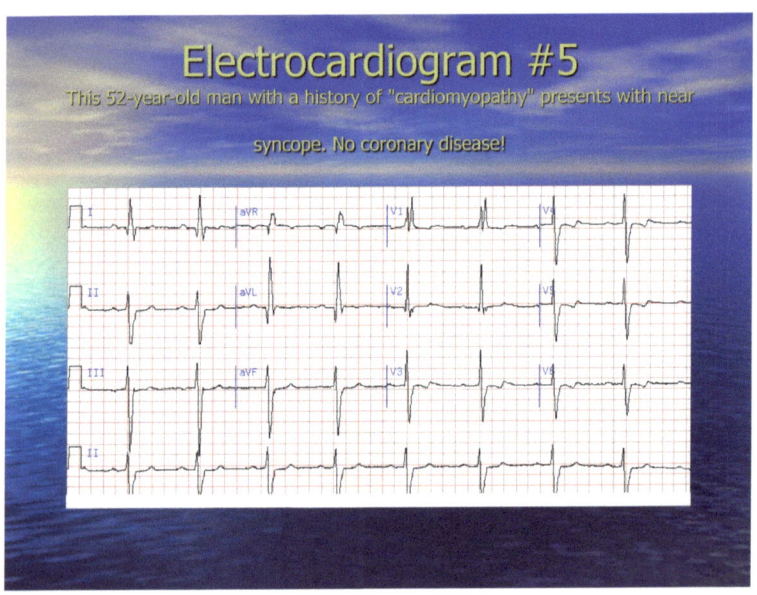

Electrocardiogram #5

This 52-year-old man with a history of "cardiomyopathy" presents with near syncope. No coronary disease!

The ECG reveals sinus rhythm with marked PR prolongation, left ventricular hypertrophy (LVH) by voltage criteria, right bundle branch block (RBBB) with left anterior fascicular block (LAFB), or "hemiblock", a prominent initial R in V1, and prominent Q waves laterally. The LVH, and the morphology of the Q's should suggest the diagnosis of hypertrophic cardiomyopathy (HCM) with asymmetric septal hypertrophy. 93% of patients with HCM have abnormal ECG's. They often have P wave evidence of left atrial abnormality, due to reduced ventricular compliance and the frequent coexistence of mitral regurgitation. Most have ECG criteria for LVH. They often have prominent Q's in the lateral leads, likely due to septal hypertrophy (the initial forces of left to right septal activation are unusually prominent. Tall broad R waves in V1 are often seen; the differential diagnosis (DDx) of this finding includes: HCM, RVH, posterior infarct, Wolff-Parkinson-White (WPW), and Duchenne's dystrophy. The absence of evidence of an inferior infarct, the absence of a short PR interval and delta waves, the left axis, and the patient's age rule out these other possibilities. In this case, there is evidence of significant conduction system disease: PR prolongation, RBBB, and LAFB. The patient later developed 2:1 heart block, and actually had improved conduction with vagal maneuvers. This improvement suggests that the PR prolongation is due to impaired infranodal conduction (as AV node proper conduction should worsen with vagal maneuvers); this type of block is worrisome for progression to high-grade heart block. The patient had an Electrophysiology study, which confirmed infranodal block. He has had improvement in his symptoms with a pacemaker. His near syncope may have been due to brady or tachyarrhythmias (tachydysrhythmias), or due to the hemodynamic consequences of his left ventricular outflow tract obstruction.

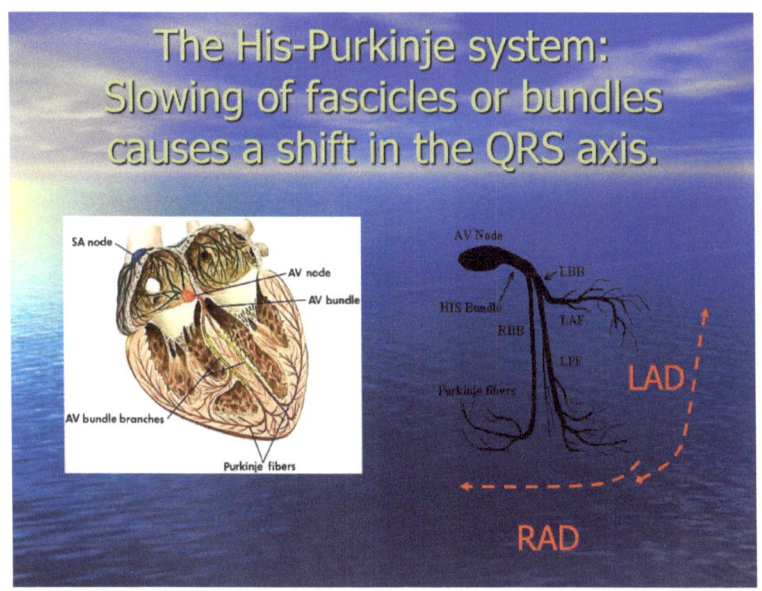
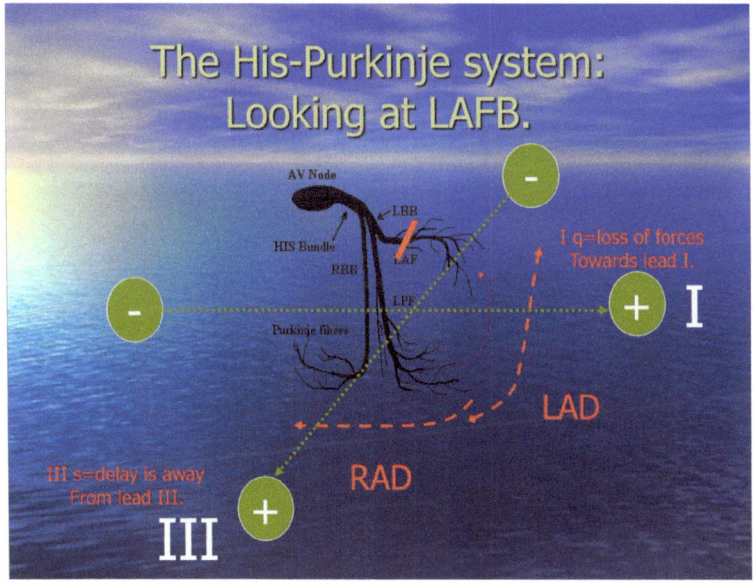

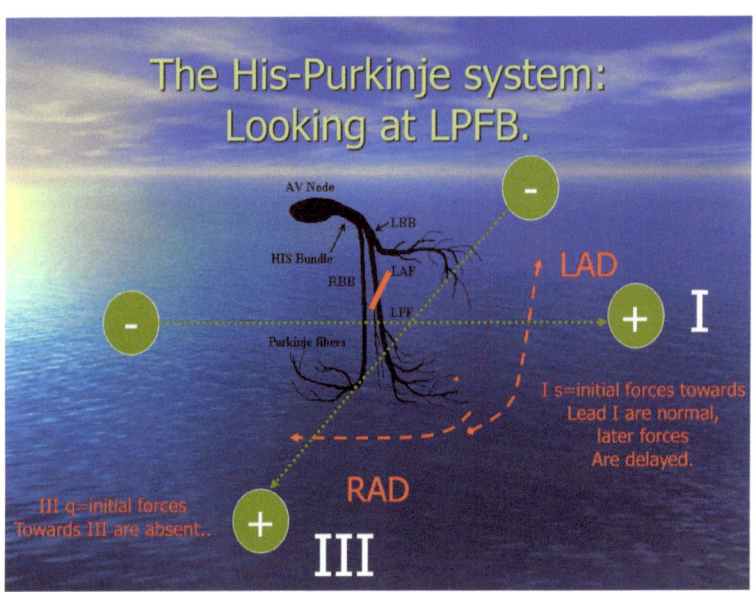

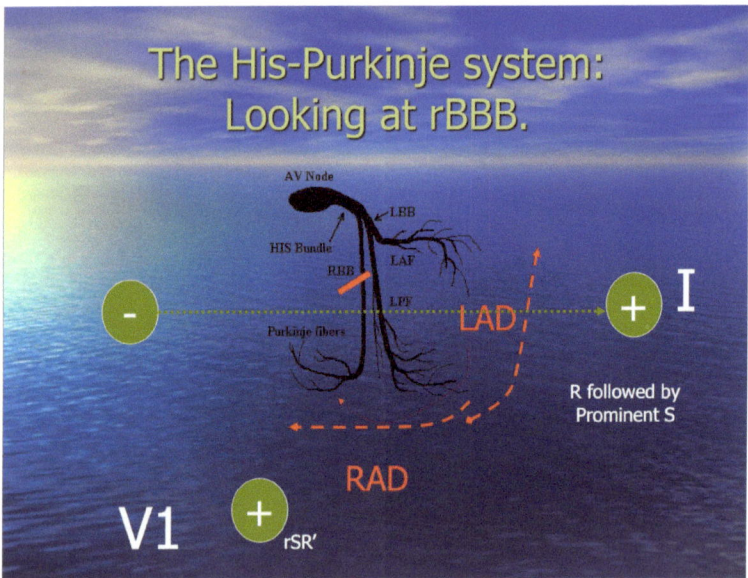

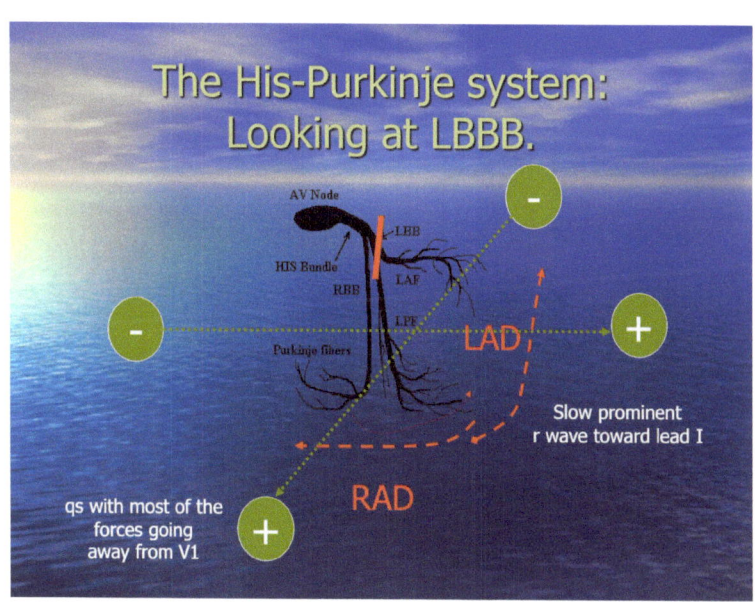

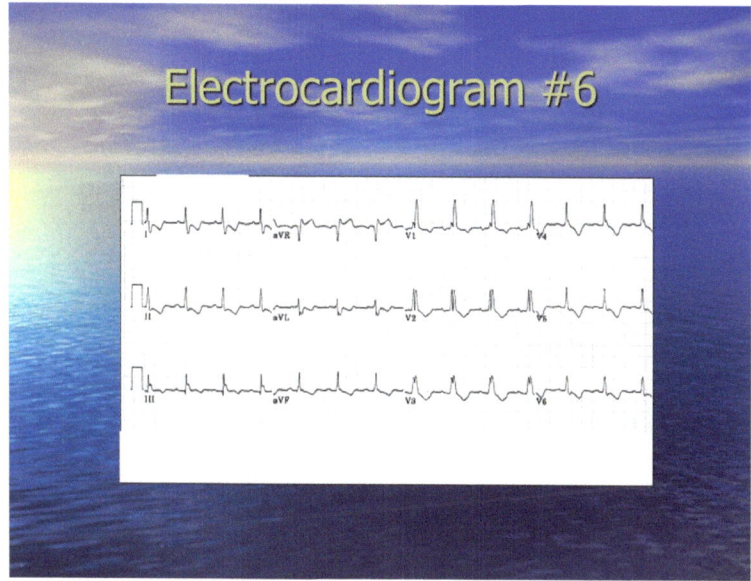

Electrocardiogram #7

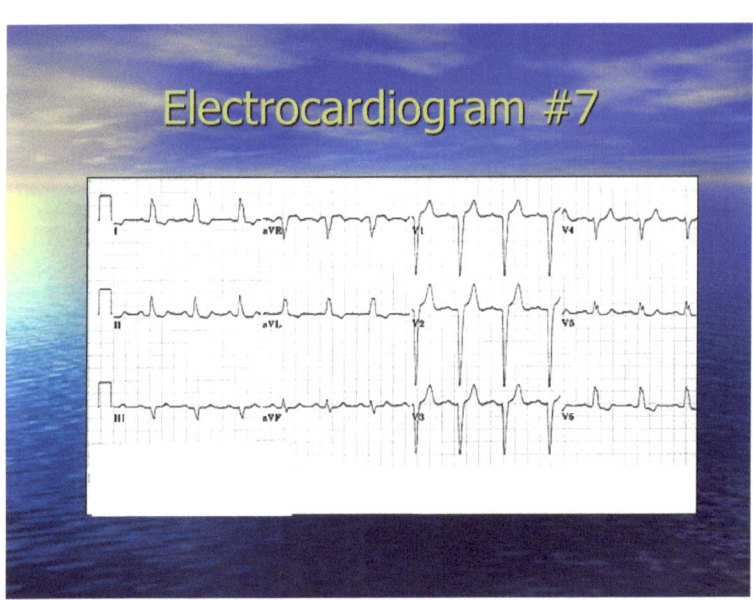

Electrocardiogram #8

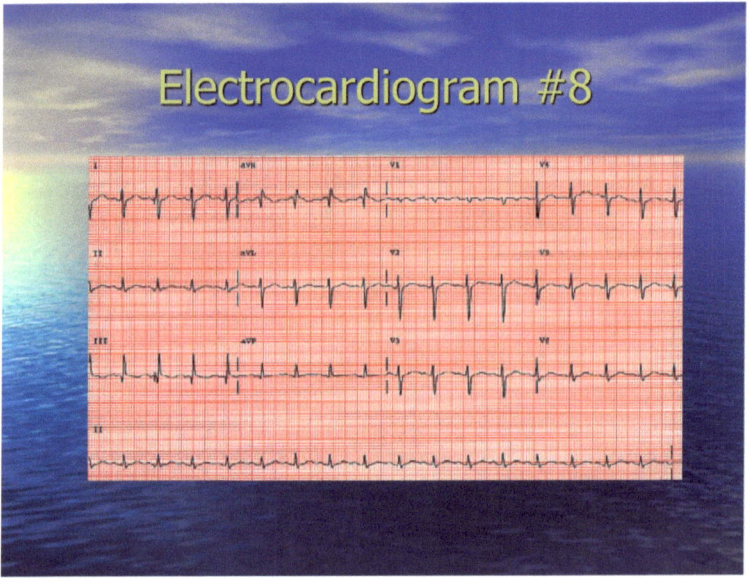

Electrocardiogram #9

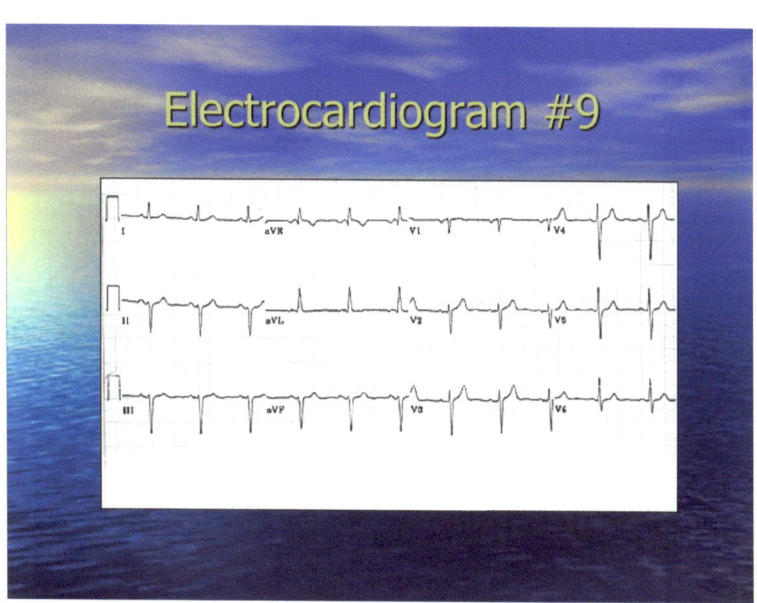

Electrocardiogram #9

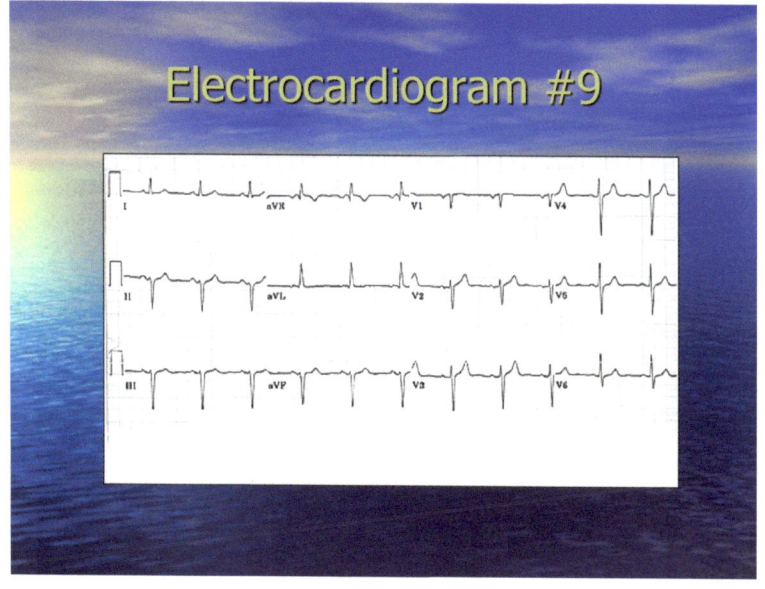

Reading Electrocardiograms

By: Dr. Richard M. Fleming
Physicist – Nuclear Cardiologist

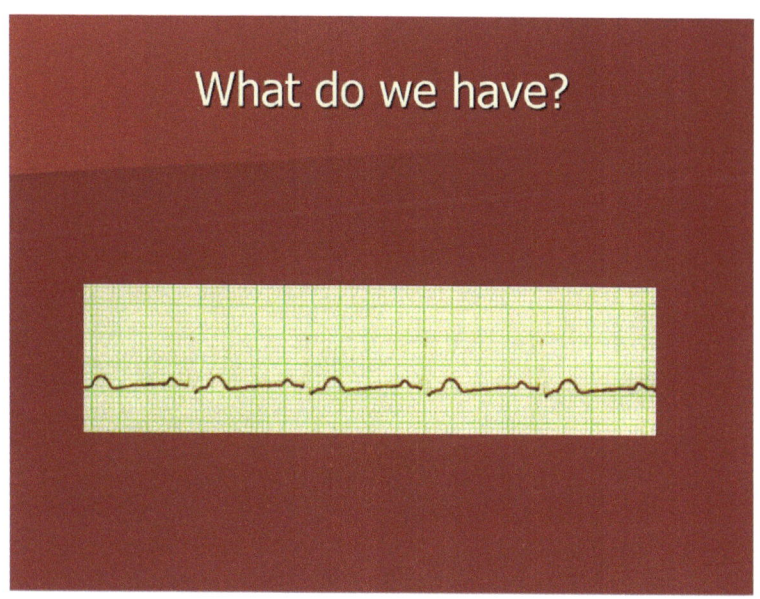

Answer: Normal Sinus Rhythm (NSR)

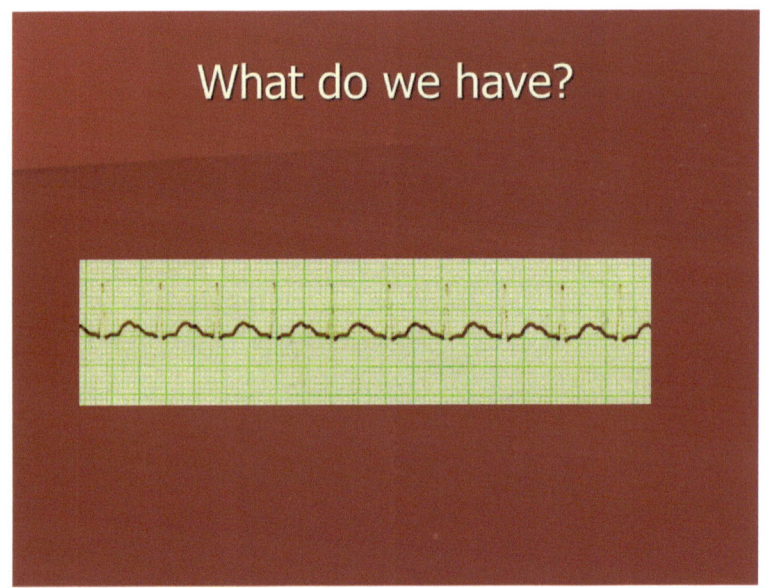

Answer: Supraventricular Tachycardia (SVT)

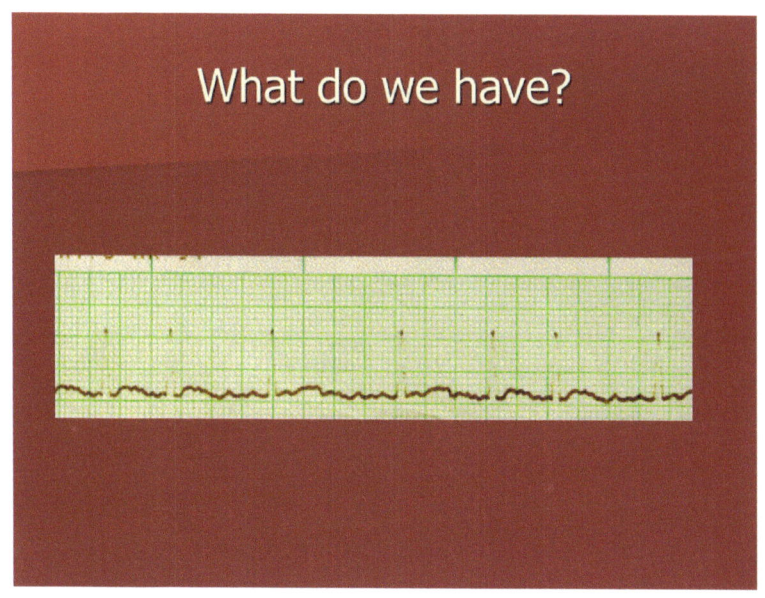

Answer: Atrial Fibrillation

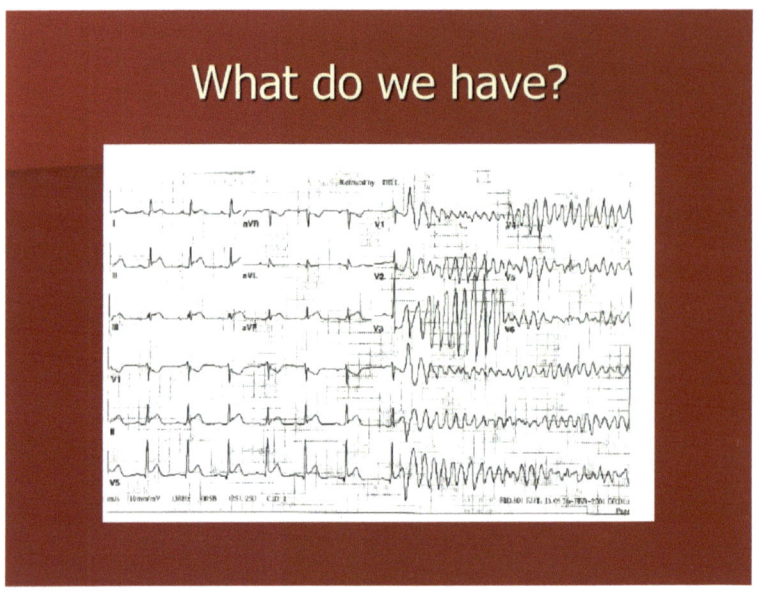

Answer: Inferior wall myocardial infarction (IWMI) with Posterior myocardial infarction (PMI) deteriorating into Ventricular Fibrillation (V Fib).

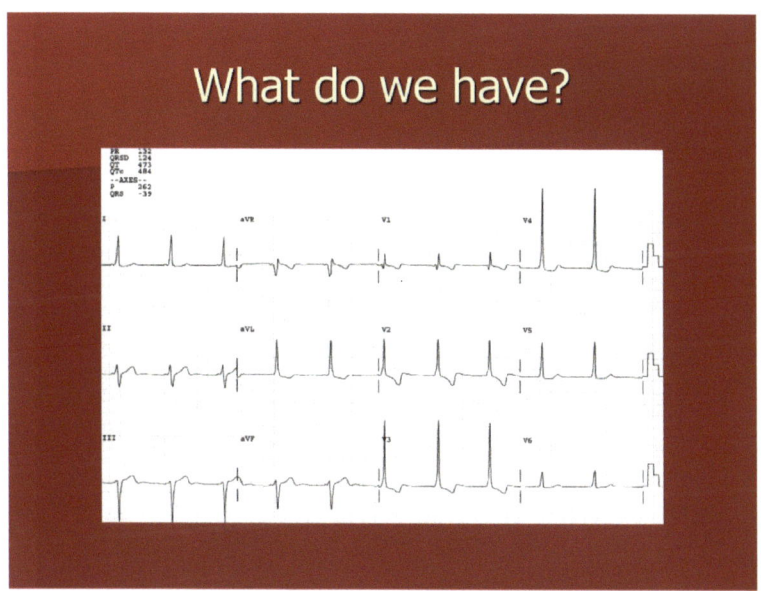

Answer: Wolff-Parkinson-White (WPW) Syndrome.

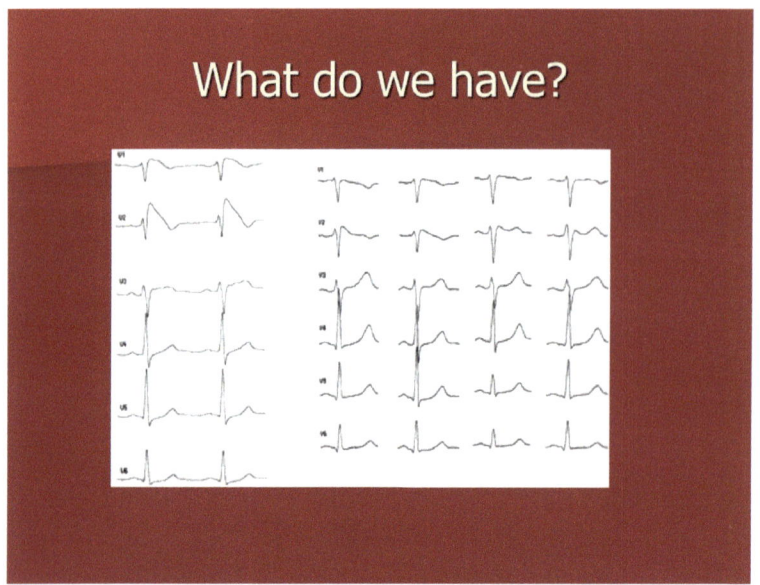

Answer: Brugada Syndrome (Genetic disorder with Sodium channel malfunction).

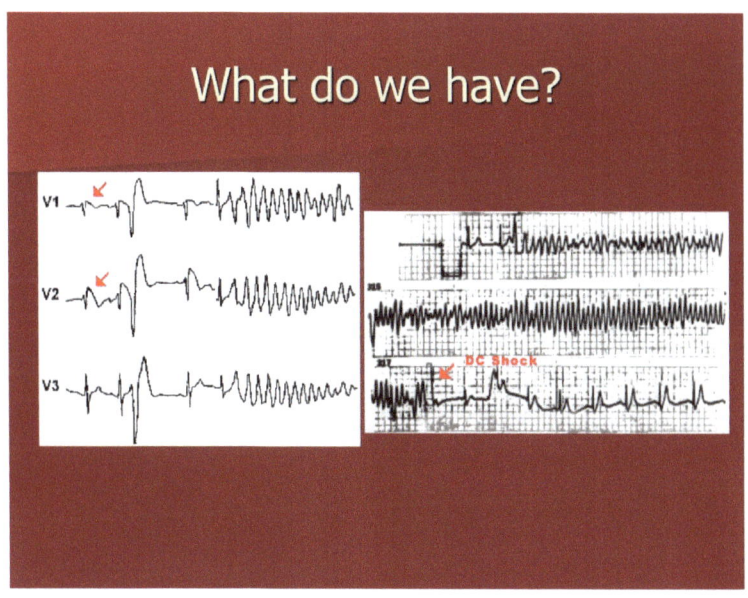

Answer: Brugada suddenly deteriorating into polymorphic ventricular tachycardia. Non-synchronized direct cardioversion defibrillation of rhythm back to sinus tachycardia.

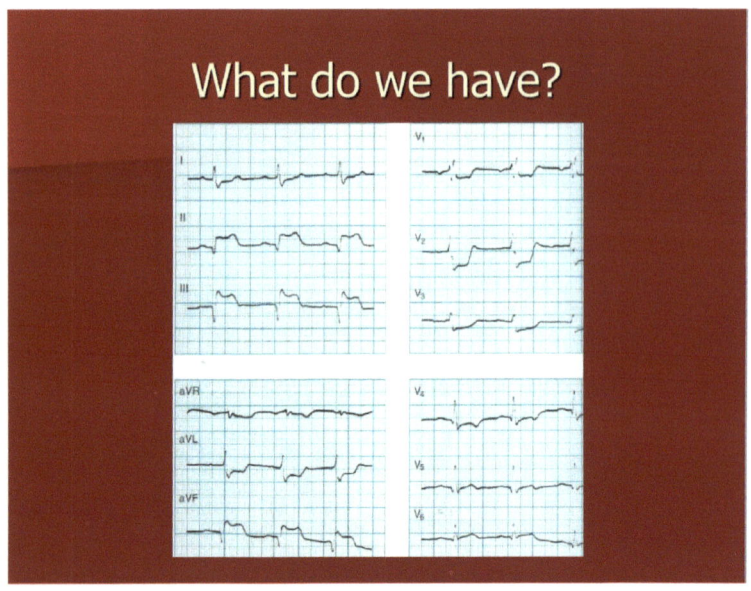

Answer: Inferior wall myocardial infarction (IWMI) and posterior myocardial infarction (PMI) with ST depression in leads V1-4.

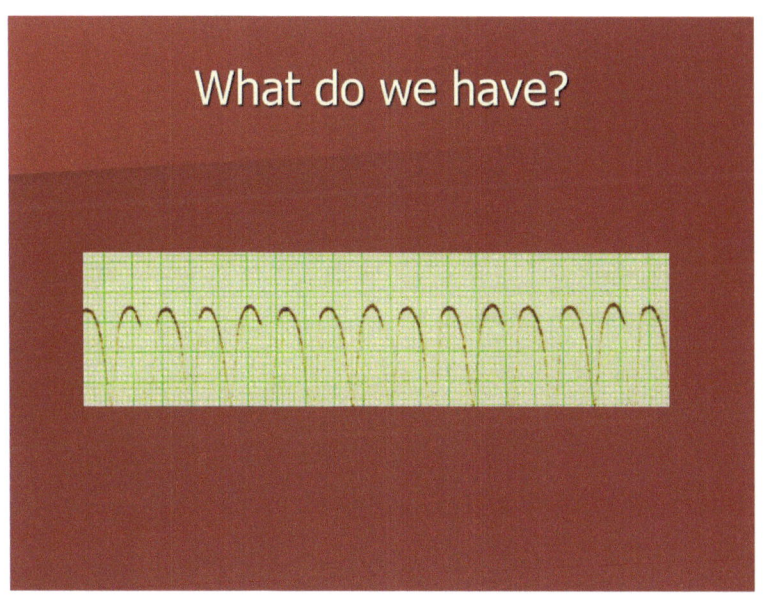

Answer: Ventricular Tachycardia

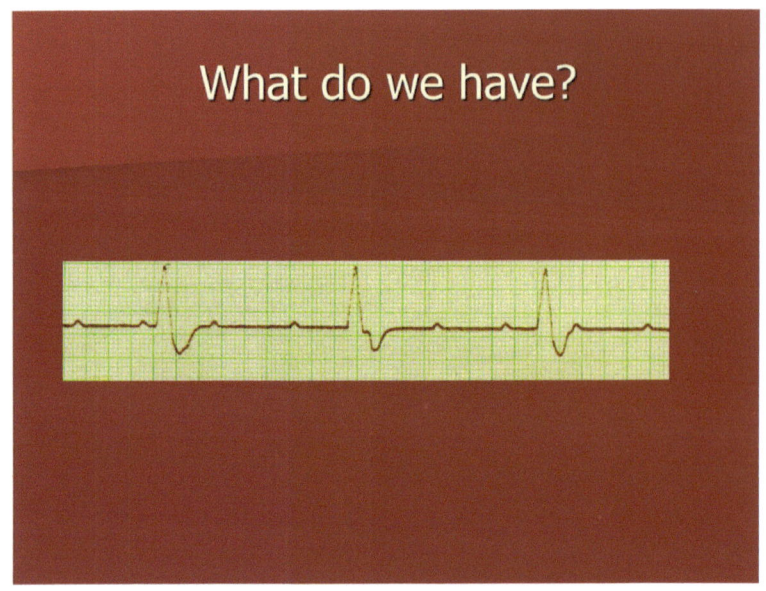

Answer: 3rd degree atrioventricular block.

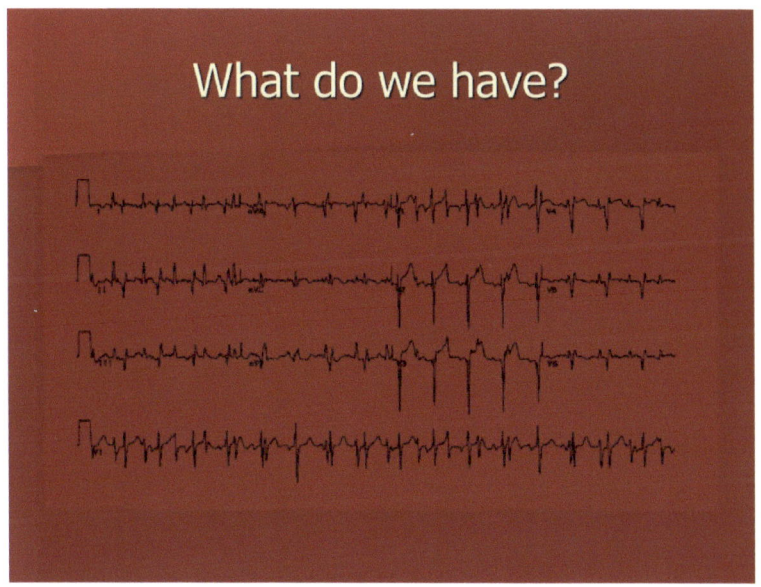

Answer: If you look for the patterns you will find two different heart rates. There are two hearts with electrical conduction following cardiac transplant.

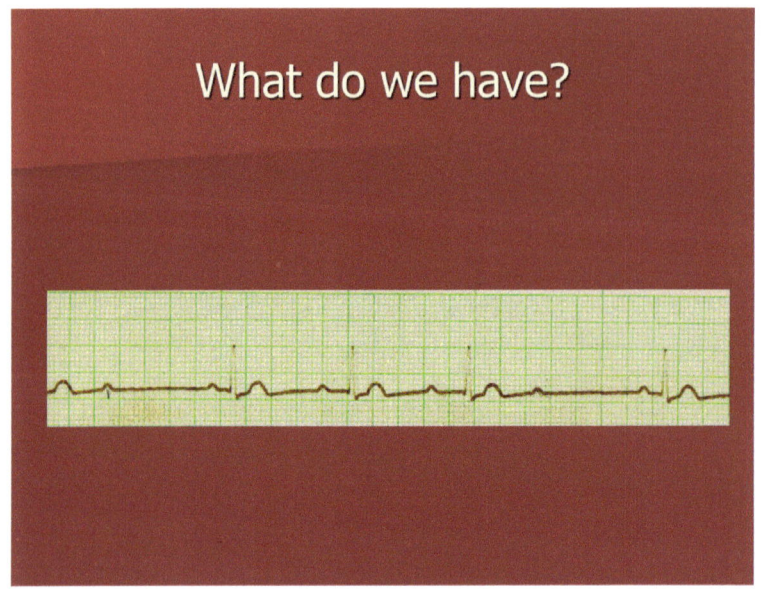

Answer: 2nd degree atrioventricular block. Mobitz II.

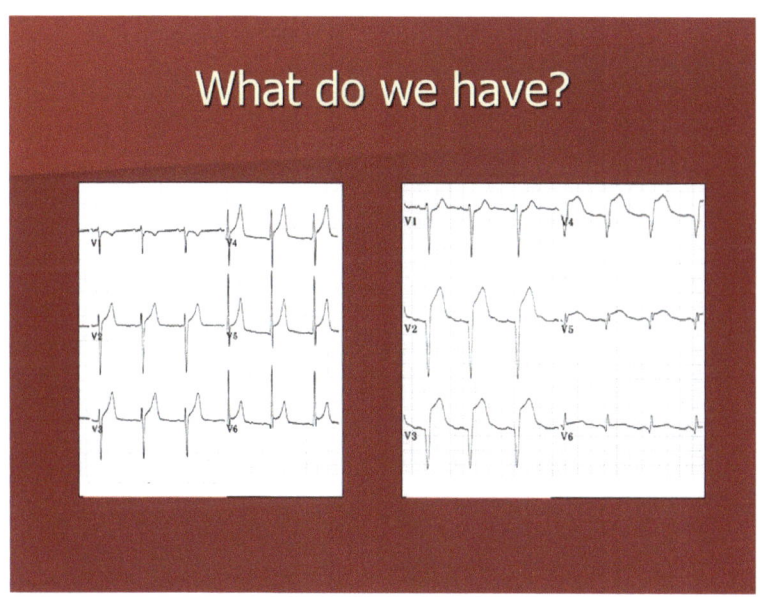

Answer: ST repolarization (concave) versus ST injury (convex).

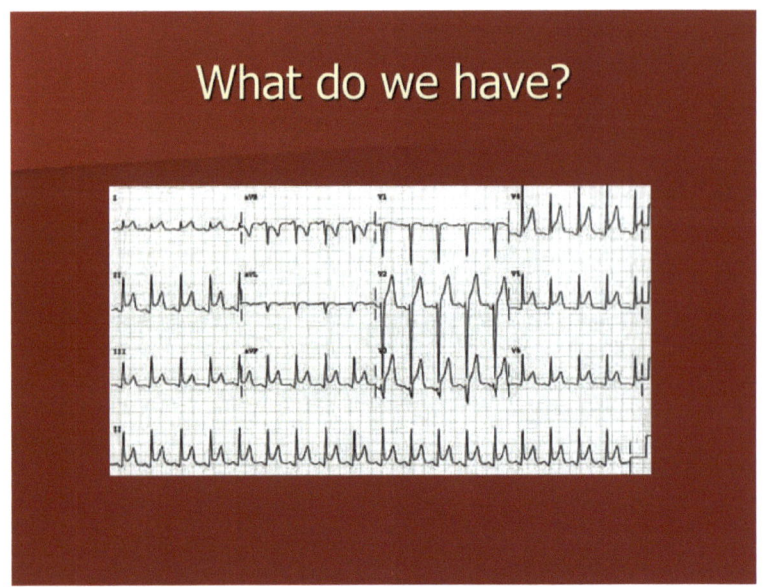

Answer: Pericarditis with diffuse ST elevation.

Wide Complex Rhythms

A variety of rhythms are seen with wide QRS complexes.

By: Dr. Richard M. Fleming
Physicist – Nuclear Cardiologist

What do you do?

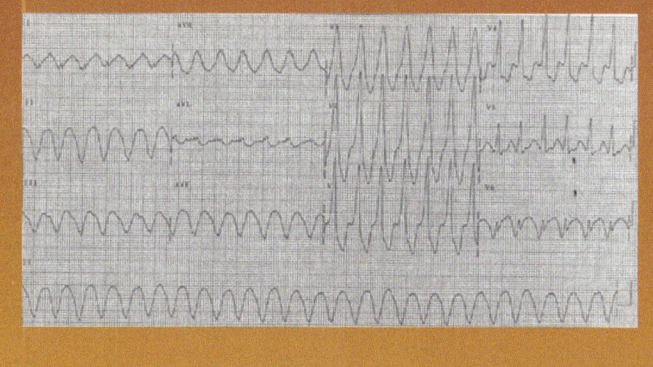

What do you do with wide complex QRS?

- Depends upon the rhythm
- The hemodynamic response
  - Is there a heart rate?
  - Is there a blood pressure?
- The clinical response
- What does cardioversion do?
  - When do you synchronize?

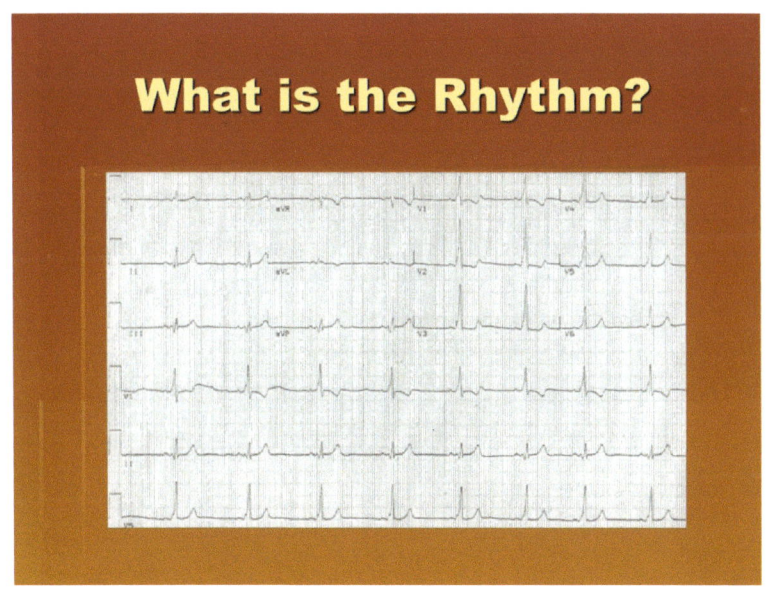

Answer: Antidromic. Conduction is traveling down an accessory pathway. The treatment of choice is DC cardioversion. Other options include Procainamide, Ibutilide, and Flecainide.

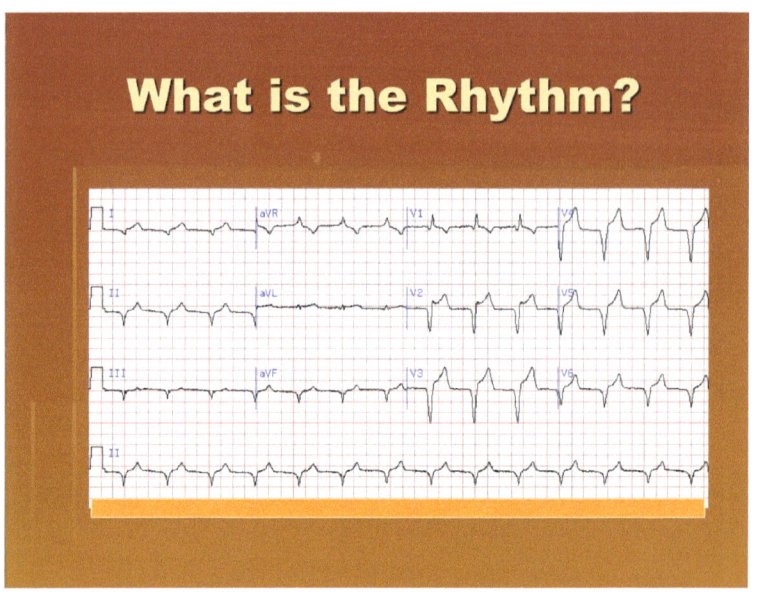

Answer: Accelerated Idioventricular Rhythm (AIVR) at 83 beats (complexes) per minute (bpm). This is a ventricular rhythm faster than the normal ventricular intrinsic rate of approximately 40 bpm and slower than ventricular tachycardia, which is defined as a ventricular rate of at least 100-120 bpm.

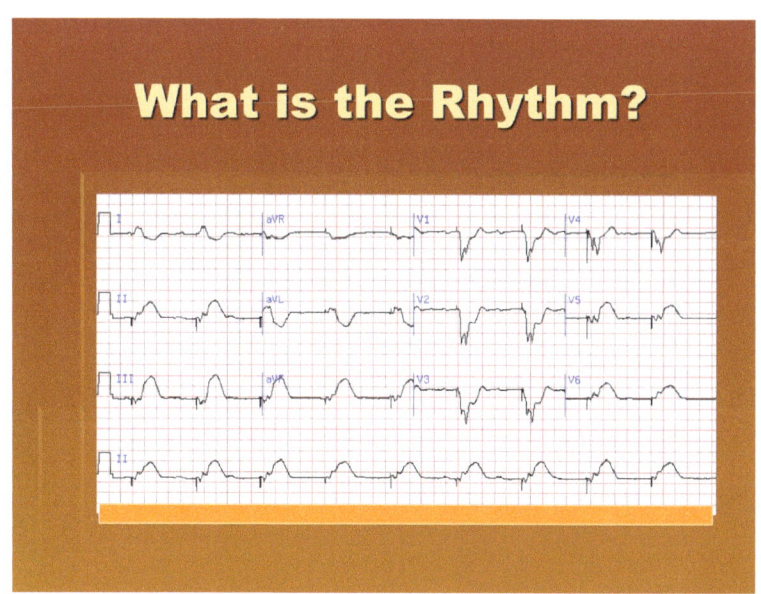

Answer: Complete heart block with ST elevation and pacer activity.

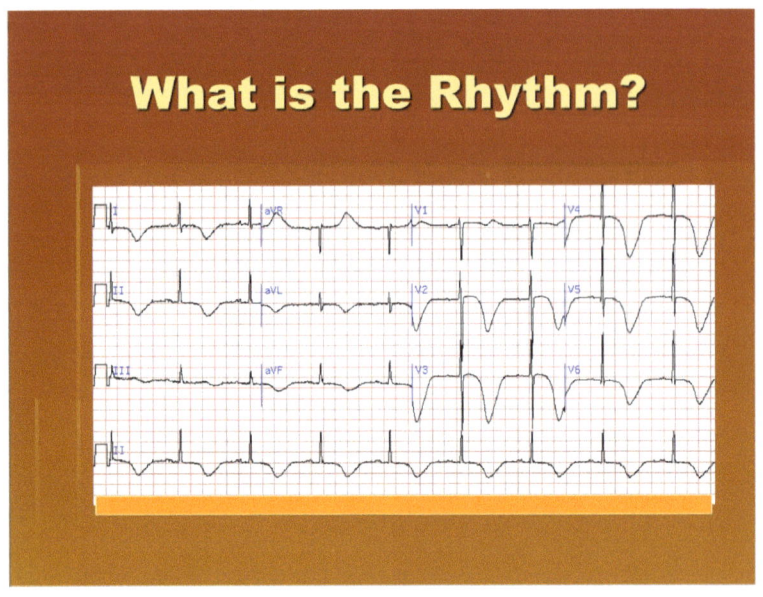

Answer: Normal sinus rhythm (NSR) with diffuse T-wave inversion. Such diffuse T-wave inversion can represent diffuse catecholamine release or triple-vessel acute coronary ischemia.

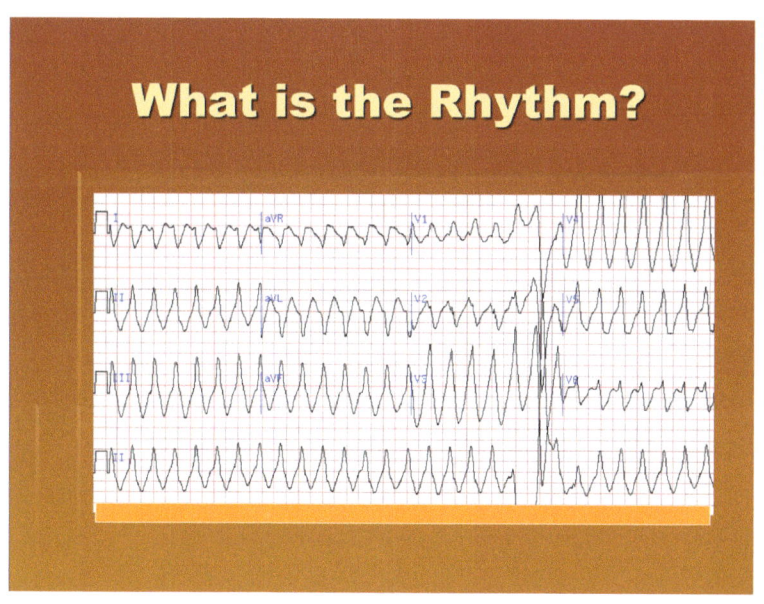

Answer: Ventricular Tachycardia (VT). The right bundle branch morphology (rBBB) tells you it is coming from the left ventricle.

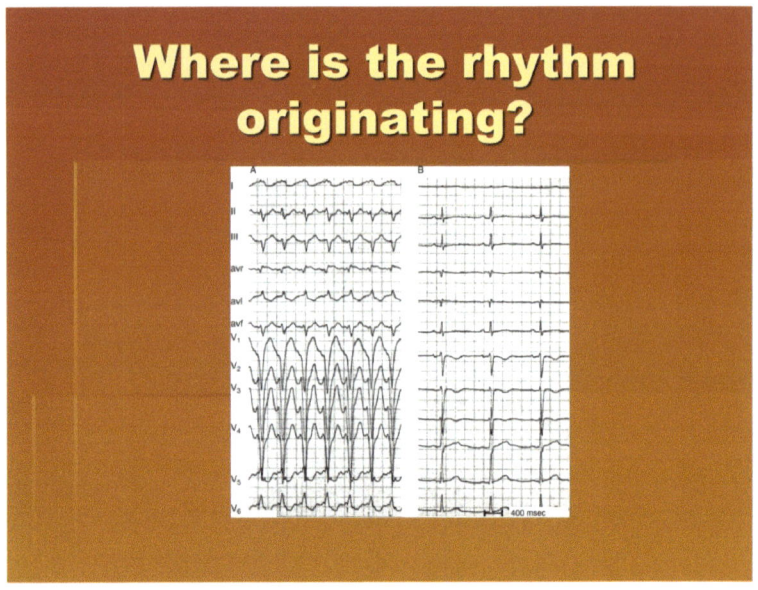

Answer: Ventricular Tachycardia (VT) in arrhythmogenic (this should actually be called dysrhythmogenic as it is not causing an absent rhythm but rather an abnormal – dys – rhythm) with right ventricular dysplasia (ARVD) origin. VT shows LBBB shape and left axis deviation indicating an origin in the apex of the right ventricle. Note also the negative T waves in V1-V3 during sinus rhythm, which is often found in ARVD.

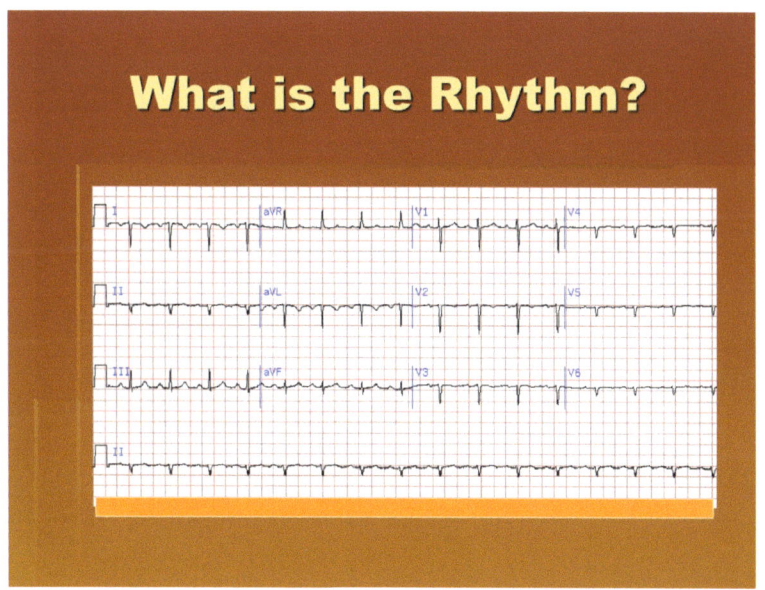

Answer: Dextrocardia. You should question lead inversion to be certain with inverted p-waves in lead I and aVL. The key to the diagnosis is the absence of R's precordially.

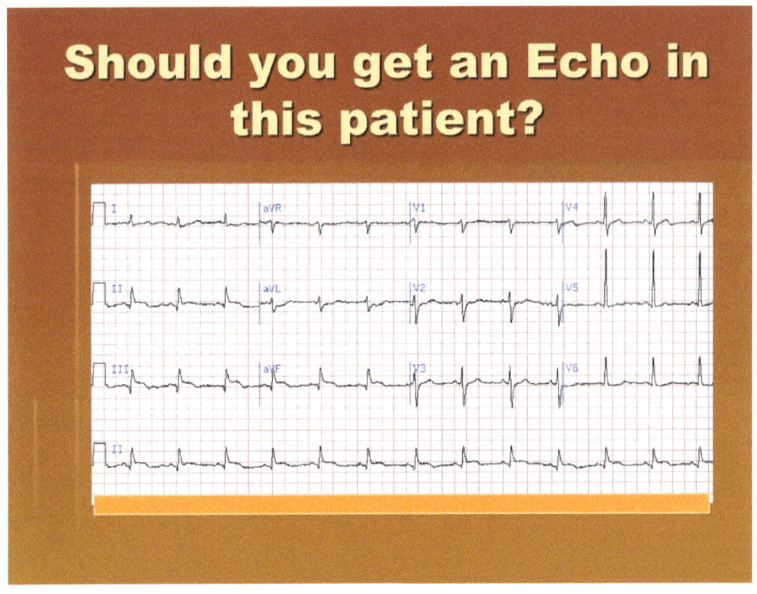

Answer: Note the inferior lead ST elevation. If there is a murmur you should consider the possibility of myocardial damage with mitral regurgitation or ventricular septal defect. The murmurs can both result from ischemia and infarction; however MR is a systolic murmur while VSD is a holosystolic murmur. An echocardiogram would aid both diagnostically and in treatment decisions.

Gaining confidence in interpreting electrocardiograms and knowing what treatment to provide to any given patient can mean the difference between life and death. This series of slides was designed to increase your level of confidence and provide you with real life examples of dysrhythmias and their treatments.

www.ingramcontent.com/pod-product-compliance
Lightning Source LLC
Chambersburg PA
CBHW040249220526
45473CB00001B/425